T0021172

Ultimate Anti-Aging Ways
Exotic Wisdom from a Japanese Doctor

Toshihito Etoh, MD, PhD

iUniverse, Inc.
New York Bloomington

Ultimate Anti-Aging Ways
Exotic Wisdom from a Japanese Doctor

Copyright © 2010 by Toshihito Etoh, MD, PhD

All rights reserved. No part of this book may be used or reproduced by any means, graphic, electronic, or mechanical, including photocopying, recording, taping or by any information storage retrieval system without the written permission of the publisher except in the case of brief quotations embodied in critical articles and reviews.

The information, ideas, and suggestions in this book are not intended as a substitute for professional medical advice. Before following any suggestions contained in this book, you should consult your personal physician. Neither the author nor the publisher shall be liable or responsible for any loss or damage allegedly arising as a consequence of your use or application of any information or suggestions in this book.

iUniverse books may be ordered through booksellers or by contacting:

iUniverse
1663 Liberty Drive
Bloomington, IN 47403
www.iuniverse.com
1-800-Authors (1-800-288-4677)

Because of the dynamic nature of the Internet, any Web addresses or links contained in this book may have changed since publication and may no longer be valid. The views expressed in this work are solely those of the author and do not necessarily reflect the views of the publisher, and the publisher hereby disclaims any responsibility for them.

ISBN: 978-1-4502-4233-2 (sc)
ISBN: 978-1-4502-4201-1 (ebk)

Library of Congress Control Number: 2010909991

Printed in the United States of America

iUniverse rev. date: 08/25/2010

Contents

Preface

For over thirty years I have been practicing medicine in Japan as a general physician in internal medicine and pediatrics. Early on in my interactions with patients I began noticing that some of them looked much younger than their true age, while others looked much older. This led me to begin searching for the reasons why there were often such remarkable discrepancies between patients' chronological ages and their physical condition. Whenever I discovered information that I thought might be helpful in solving this riddle, I made careful note of it. From these observations I have developed some very successful strategies for slowing down the aging process, not only in the body, but also in the mind. Whenever I have advised my patients to do these practices and exercises, all of them have succeeded in becoming younger looking and younger thinking. Based on these experiences, a strong desire to share this knowledge about anti-aging has grown in me.

Ever since ancient times, the Japanese have had many techniques for keeping fit and living longer. Today, the cities and the countryside are filled with very active elderly people. In 2006 the life expectancy for Japanese woman was over eighty-six, and for Japanese men, seventy-nine. I really think that's amazing! In the future, people from other countries may look forward to living this long.

Although we can't escape from death, in this book I offer several ideas and techniques to help you stay young as long as possible as well as maintain a high quality of life. Fortunately, nobody has to invest lots of money and time to put these techniques and ideas into practice. Above all, this book was designed for practical use. If you do at least some of these practices and exercises, they will help you to combat aging as well as keep fit. In addition, if you were worried about your weight, you will benefit from this book. Of course, it will be up to you to decide which exercises to do.

By following the ideas contained in this book, you can improve your fitness and your well-being. I invite you to read on.

Acknowledgments

This book could not have been written without the extreme patience and love of my wife, Mieko Etoh, and my sons, Hitoshi Etoh and Tsutomu Etoh. I really appreciate their help.

My special thanks goes to Martin Skrypnyk, who edited the entire book, including the references. More than that, Martin has been a wonderful support in giving me useful suggestions for this task based on his experience in Japan. My thanks also to Greg Goodbeer, who first edited the tile and the preface. Again, a special thanks to Ellen Peppard, who not only made a great effort to draw all the illustrations but also assisted in the improvement of my writing skills. Samantha Stroh Bailey, Nathan Baker, and Roberto Addari provided much knowledge about publishing. I was lucky to have been a student at pacific Language Institute (PLI), in Toronto, where I studied English with many good teachers and friends. I appreciate all of them.

Chapter 1: Knowing Yourself

Have you ever thought about who you are? Have you ever wondered if you truly exist? Well, you do, and you really are reading this book and breathing the air on the earth. There is no other person like you on this earth. This is a fact. You are unique. You are one of the precious creatures that nature has produced. You are the cutting edge in human evolution. Your existence and life is a miracle! That being the case, I hope you will recognize just how wonderful you are.

If you ask yourself who you are, it might be difficult for you to answer immediately. How deeply does one know or understand oneself? In Japan, some people ponder this question while sitting peacefully, like a frog. This practice is called zazen, which is a sitting meditation essential to Zen Buddhism. In this book, I do not intend to force you to do zazen. However, it is extremely important to know and understand yourself if you want to stay young and fit. The practice of meditation will help you to achieve that self-awareness. Unless you know enough about your present self, you won't be able to see the change compared to your past self or imagine your future self.

Knowing yourself is the first step in combating the aging process. Your body and mind have been changing day by day for the entire course of your life. The cells that make up your body have been replaced by new ones again and again. Of course, you know there is much difference between the past and present in both your body and mind. Like a couple figure skating, your body and mind are in a close relationship, and they are constantly changing form. Knowing yourself means knowing both your body and your mind.

When you look in a mirror, you may see an overweight body and wrinkles on your face, both clear signs of aging. Looking at yourself honestly might be stressful. However, it is necessary for you to have the courage to accept your present self. It might also force you recognize the fact you have to act to lose those extra pounds. It is time to make a decision!

As for the mind, it can seem a little bit more difficult to know, as there is no mirror you can hold up to it. However, you should not let this discourage you. There is a simple way for you to get to know your mind. Remember the ambitions and hopes of your youth? Whether vivid in your memory or tucked away in some corner and slightly dusty, you should try to reconnect with these delightful things that may have been lost long ago. If you think of them, the sense of vitality you had in that long forgotten day of your youth may come back to you. It might be the memory of the hottest passion. That is not to say that you should regret its disappearance, however. Its disappearance does not matter. You do not have to regret it because now you have a chance to find a possible cause of suffering in your mind. It is more important to think about how to get rid of that suffering in the mind than to regret the past. It is worth finding a way out of the suffering in order to have a more delightful future. In other words, there is not only hope but also a shining way to the future in front of you, regardless of your previous life.

You should not be afraid of walking toward the future. Have confidence in yourself. You have to remind yourself that your existence and life is a miracle. Moreover, you have survived an environment that has been drastically and restlessly changing. You have enough power to improve yourself *by yourself.* Encourage yourself! Trust yourself! Use chapters 2 through 7 as a guide, but if you want to stay youthful, you have to take matters into your own hands.

Chapter 2: Realization of the Soul

A s I've said, both our bodies and our minds are changing every day. However, I think that there must be something that remains unchanged throughout our life. The Greek philosopher Plato regarded everything in the world as an essence that has a permanent and indestructible existence outside of space and time. According to him, every individual, without exception, has some kind of unchanged and indestructible spirit that he called "the soul." The soul is something essential, the core of your being. By becoming aware of the soul, we wake up to the fact that we are a part of the cosmos. Without doubt, your awareness of the soul is one of the most important factors in your attitude toward aging because the soul is beyond time and therefore never changes. Not only do you have to be aware of its presence, but you also have to take care of it.

How can you become aware of your soul? I think that one uses what I like to call a "seventh sense" to detect the existence of the soul. This is different from a sixth sense, which seems to be a gut feeling. When we make a decision, we often use our gut feeling instead of logical thinking. For example, when we want to listen to a CD, we may choose classical music one day and pop or jazz another day. In this example, our gut feeling forces us to make an unconscious decision based on reasons obscure to us. It is kind of an inner voice.

The seventh sense is much different from the other six senses. Although you have had a seventh sense from birth, you may not recognize it yet. The following exercise will help you recognize this sense, thereby bringing about an awareness of your soul. As crazy as it may seem, try to have a conversation with a big tree. It should be easy to find one either in a park (well, maybe you don't want people to see you talking to a tree) or in the woods. After you choose the tree, you should wrap your arms around it tightly and try to communicate with it in silence. It has been around longer than you have, so you can talk about the past with it. "Do you remember what was happening around you thirty years ago?" you might ask. Or perhaps you might say, "My friend, can you listen to my life story?" You should have a conversation about what has happened to you throughout your life. Of course, the tree can't speak. However, as you continuously attempt to communicate with the tree, you will begin to felling a sense of connectedness with it. Do this as often as necessary. The tree has been living on our planet just as you have, and it is part of nature just as you are. And in Plato's sense, it has a soul. If you leave yourself open to this possibility, you will realize something delightful when you make the effort to communicate with nature.

Here is another great exercise you can try. First, lie on your back in bed and close your eyes. Make sure that it's quiet and the lights are off. Relax all of your muscles. (Actually, this is not so easy to do, so don't get discouraged if it takes a bit of patience to get the hang of it.) One way of making sure that your muscles are loose and relaxed is to flex and tighten all of them without moving any part of your body and then suddenly let go and relax. In every part of your body, from head to foot, you should repeatedly practice this. For example, gradually tense up your left arm without moving it, and keep it this way for a moment. Then, immediately release all the tension from the left arm. If you repeat this procedure two or three times, you will not feel any weight in your left arm at all.

In the same way, do this with your right arm, and then continue until you have succeeded in releasing the tension from every part of your body (face, neck, shoulder, arm, hand, belly, back, leg, foot). Eventually, you will feel weightless, as if you are floating in space. This is a state or condition conducive to self-awareness, as it allows you to sense the self without the burden of feeling the body.

At first it will take a lot of time to get into a completely relaxed, peaceful, and comfortable condition. However, once you do, this exercise will help keep you youthful in both body and mind because you can face the soul in yourself through it. If you continue this practice for about twenty minutes at least twice a week, you will reach a stage where you will feel as if you are being hugged lovingly by the earth itself, just as your mother held you when you were a newborn baby. It is not only a time of self-awareness, but also a time to truly nourish your soul.

Chapter 3: Awakening of Sleeping Memory in Every Cell

In this chapter, I will show you how a combination of meditation, focus, and breathing can combat aging. The basis of this attractive innovation was established by a Japanese doctor named Shinzaburou Shioya. Seeking health and fitness, he created a method that he called *seishin chousoku hou*. Through its practice, he could still enjoy playing golf twice a week even at ninety-five years of age.

What is *seishin chousoku hou*? It is a method based on a combination of meditation and breathing. *Seishin* means "relief from an evil mind." He said that if we seek this relief, we will live a peaceful and happy life without harming anyone else.

According to his explanation, *chousoku hou* refers to a method of breathing by which we can inhail the maximum amount of energy in the air into every cell in our bodies. He claimed that we could live a long and healthy life if we continuously practiced this method, which is actually based on the belief that a human is made up of about eight trillion cells, each of which have both intention and memory. (Here, memory is not the same as DNA.) In other words, his belief comes from the idea that both intention and memory exist not only in the brain but also in the other cells in the body. His idea closely links to my idea that the soul is indestructible and exists in every cell in the body equally. Actually, I think both the intention and memory of each cell might be a part of the soul.

Dr. Shioya suffered from a urinary disorder, which he was able to cure entirely through *seishin chousoku hou.* No medication was used. In order to wake up the sleeping memory in his every cell, he had been visualizing the relief of his condition while practicing his original breathing method every day. After one month he was able to urinate normally. He claimed that during this practice he never anticipated the cure, but simply imagined his body functioning smoothly, and that it was very important to visualize the predictable result in order to make his wish come true.

I think that his method is brilliant. However, both patience and continuous practice are necessary. I've tried to add to this method while retaining the breathing practice.

Let's start with the breathing. In this procedure you have to inhale and exhale through your nose. First, you take a deep breath, feeling the air filling up and expanding your lungs. Second, you need to hold your breath for one or two seconds as a slow transition. Third, you exhale from your nose little by little. While exhaling, you need to visualize the air slowly moving out from the bottom of your belly. Finally, after exhaling, take a short breath. This sequence of breathing may be done in either a sitting or lying position, but it should be done for more than ten minutes, once or twice a day, with your eyes closed and your hands clasped together resting on the lap.

Although Dr. Shioya claimed that the combination of breathing and meditation could cure illness, I will tell you how meditation, which I originally developed, can help you stay youthful. In fact, this method can also help you lose weight. Fortunately, I have had several successful cases of people who lost about eighteen pounds in body weight after consistent practice for only two months. This success seemed to be due to a change in metabolism. As we age our metabolism slows, and as a result, we tend to gain weight. However, if we can raise our metabolism through meditation, our body weight will naturally decrease, despite eating regularly. That is to say, it is extremely important to force every cell to remind both the body and the mind of your youth. Moreover, in order to remind both the body and the mind of your youth, it is extremely useful to awaken the sleeping memory in every cell through the meditation. How can you awaken the sleeping memory in every cell? I will show you an easy way to do so.

Do you remember the songs that were popular when you were young? For example, if you are around sixty years old, you likely remember the Carpenters' music, especially "Top of the World" or "Sing." During meditation, try to remember the songs, and imagine yourself listening to them. Moreover, you need to actually listen to the music in your mind, without the aid of CDs or MP3s. Of course, it does not need to be the Carpenter's music. Any song you listened to in your youth will work. By doing this you can evoke the memory of not only your younger self but also the environment you used to live in. Eventually, you can identify yourself as a young man or woman in your own mind. If you practice this combination of meditation and breathing every day, your body and mind undergo an amazing transformation, helping you stay youthful.

Chapter 4: Walking and Posture

During the course of my thirty-four years as a doctor, I have seen lots of patients, from newborn to centenarian. My experience has taught me how important walking is in our life. Let's think about the stages of our life. We mostly lie at birth, crawl and stand at one year of age, and lie in old age and death. However, walking occupies a good portion of our lives. We should be paying attention to not only the amount of time we spend walking but the manner in which we walk. Have you ever thought about what kind of walking is best for your health?

Good walking involves taking long strides, landing on our heels, keeping our back straight, and swinging our arms in a synchronized movement with our legs. However, it is difficult to concentrate on these movements all the time, so I wondered how I could make good walking easier. Eventually, I found the solution. I realized that the center of gravity in the body is critical because walking is a movement against gravity. If there were no gravity, we would never walk.

But where is the center of gravity located in the body? It exists at about the level of the fifth lumber vertebra, which corresponds to the central portion of the lower back. By paying attention to the position of this area of the back, you can easily improve your walking posture. The key is keeping this part of your body the center of gravity. In practicing this, your walking can improve remarkably without having to think of all the actions involved in the activity. I once advised a class of elementary students to try this for one year. Not only did their posture improve but their athletic ability increased. Again, you should focus on keeping the lower central portion of your back as the center of your gravity whenever you walk. You will not only feel healthier but look younger walking with a straight back rather than hunched over.

We take standing upright for granted, and yet it is an extremely rare act for other animals to perform. However, our posture can't help but deteriorate under gravity as time goes by. As a result, we tend to hunch over as we age until finally we can't get up by ourselves. If your posture is bad, then, without doubt, you look older than your real age. In contrast, if your posture is good, you look younger than your real age. In addition, a bad posture may cause a rapid decrease in athletic ability. Throughout life, you need to maintain a good posture.

The jaw joint, spine, and pelvis are essential components in helping us to stand upright. If one component suffers, the others suffer as well. Don't forget that humans are vertebrates!

First, let's look at the jaw. Your jaw works hard whenever you are chewing. When you are dealing with a stressful situation, you may notice that your jaw is often tensed. You may also grind in your sleep; there again it is the jaw that is being stressed. This area of the body generally gets paid little heed, but it is one that is often overworked. But what should you do to relax it? There are two approaches to the problem. One is to intentionally yawn, which not only makes the muscle attached to the jaw relax but also relieves the jaw joint itself from stiffness. You may have seen images of lions yawning. One of the main reasons for doing this is to relax the jaw and the muscle attached to it because they have to use their jaws to attack prey. The behavior of the lion teaches us how to take care of our jaws. Try yawning intentionally!

Another useful practice, which was established by Mr. Ichinami, a famous dental technician in Japan, involves opening your mouth and bridging either a chopstick or a pencil between the corners of the mouth while sitting on a chair (Fig. 1). It is very important not to bite down on the chopstick or the pencil, as the purpose of this is to relax your jaw. It should be done for ten minutes two or three times a day. It is so easy, and all you need is a chopstick or a pencil.

Now think about what would happen if your spine didn't work well. Like the rest of the body, the spine deteriorates over the years, but you can protect it with a simple and easy exercise. Lying on your back in bed, first turn your head to the right, stretching both the right arm and leg while bending the left arm and leg (Fig. 2). You should keep that position for five minutes. Then, you turn your head to the left and repeat the exercise on the opposite side for another five minutes (Fig. 3).

The pelvis is also essential in maintaining a good posture, but its position tends to shift in later years. To avoid this, there is another easy exercise that can be done in bed. First, you should put the back of your right hand in your left palm (Fig. 4). Then, put both hands under the head and bend the left leg, placing your foot over the right knee (Fig. 5). You should keep that position for five minutes. Then, putting the back of your left hand in your right palm (Fig. 6), repeat this position on the opposite side (Fig. 7). Daily practice will improve your posture remarkably. And a good posture keeps you fit and youthful.

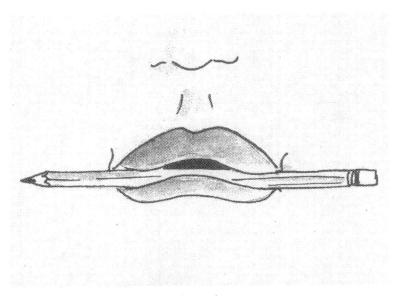

(Fig. 1)

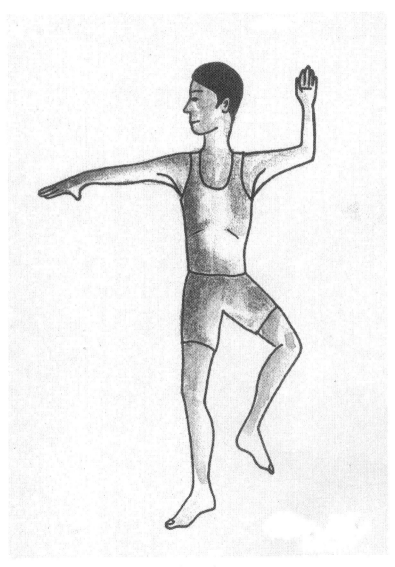

(Fig. 2)

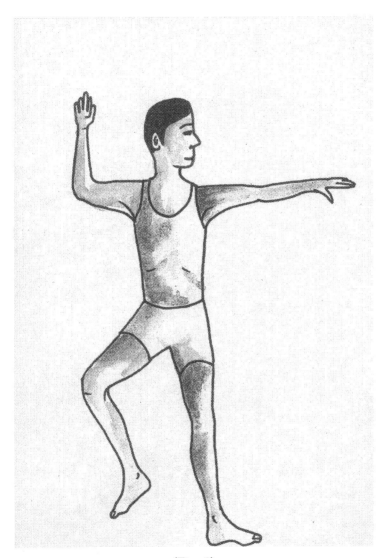

(Fig. 3)

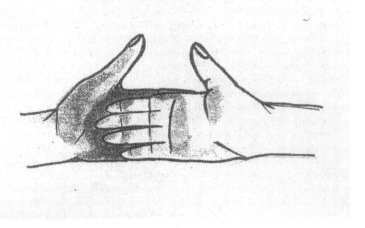

(Fig. 4)

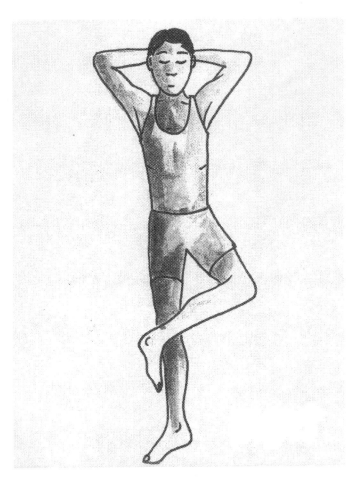

(Fig. 5)

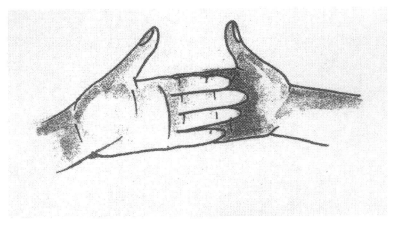

(Fig. 6)

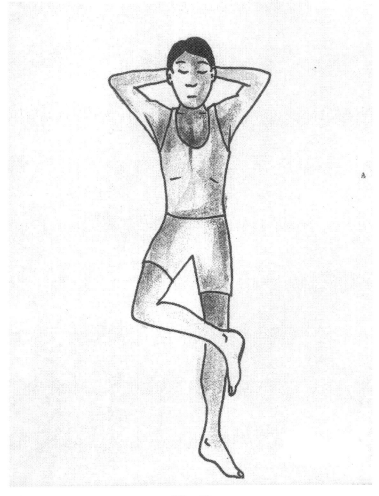

(Fig. 7)

Chapter 5: Brain, Tongue, and the Senses of Sight and Touch

The human brain is divided into two sides, or hemispheres, the right and the left. In general, the left hemisphere specializes in controlling language, while the right specializes in using information received from the senses: sight, sound, smell, touch, and taste. However, the right and left hemispheres do not work in isolation but rather cooperate in all human activity. Lots of information, which has been received from the above senses, contributes to human activity like thinking and speaking. From the point of view, the human brain is surely stimulated by such senses as well as by thinking and speaking. In this chapter, I will show you how to shape up the brain with our tongue or senses of sight and touch.

Humans often take language and speech for granted, but these skills developed over much of the course of human evolution.

Needless to say, we rely on speech to communicate with each other. And after speech, reading and writing followed. Have you ever thought what there needs to use when we speak? Well, nobody can speak without a tongue. Our tongues have evolved along with our brain in a close relationship. Moreover, during the days from infant to child, we become to get the ability of speaking through daily tongue training.

On the other hand, we can also see the connection between the brain and movement of the tongue in the case of a woman with a balance disorder, which was reported by Dr. Doidge, author of *The Brain that Changes Itself.* She couldn't walk due to the dizziness she would feel upon standing—a result of having lost the function of her inner ear, which helps to maintain balance. However, she was eventually able to stand and walk using her tongue, in which had been implanted a plastic strip with small electrodes connected to her brain.

We might be able to stimulate our brain with our tongues. Like everything else in the human body, the brain ages and slows down with age. Therefore we need to protect its functions if we are to stay young and fit. I think that the more you move your tongue, the more your brain is stimulated. But how can you exercise your tongue? Try sticking it out and writing your name or a short sentence ("I'm fine and still young," for example) in the air, using only the tip of your tongue like a pen, and without moving your head. This action looks silly, but it may be very useful in stimulating the brain. If you do this around ten times a day, I believe you will succeed in maintaining or even raising the ability of your brain.

What about our senses of sight and touch? What can we do to keep them " in shape" and at the same time stimulate the brain?

Animals need eyes for many reasons, but they developed the sense of sight mainly as aid to catching prey. As a result, the eye has to quickly respond to the rapid movement of prey. Since we are animals ourselves, our eyes have served a similar purpose. By means of detecting movement, our eyes need to move both widely and quickly. Basically, they are likely not to be created to see or detect anything without moving. From the point of view, whether we are reading a book, or working online for a long time, our eyes are engaging in extraordinary work, with which our visual ability gets down eventually.

In order to avoid the visual dysfunction associated with aging, we need to widely see various portions as quickly as possible as well. One exercise is to repeatedly move your eyes left and right, and up and down, as quickly as possible while you are looking at the sky without moving your head. This practice should be done for fifteen seconds several times a day. The other is to, sometimes, alternately turn your head back and forth to looking back over each shoulder while walking. At that time, you will have to move your eyes quickly to see both the right side and the left side alternately. If you get into the habit of doing this exercise while daily walking, naturally, such rapid movement of your eyes will stimulate your brain and also keep you safe from dangers behind you, such as rushing motorists or bicyclists.

Without your sense of touch, life would be more difficult than you think. If you were blind, you would not walk without using the sense of touch. Small children feel their mother's love when she touches or embraces them. The skin is essential, acting as a conduit for this sensation.

In Japan, the traditional way to stimulate the skin is called *kampumasatsu*. *Kampumasatsu* involves rubbing the skin with a dry towel. This is done on all areas of the body except for the head. You should take care not to rub the skin too hard. It should feel comfortable because the purpose is to stimulate the brain by activating the sense of touch. This practice is especially useful if it is done before bathing. (Those suffering from a skin disease should avoid this practice.)

Chapter 6: Breathing

nimal means "breathing creature" in Latin. Nobody can live without breathing. We get oxygen from the air and produce carbon dioxide as a waste through breathing. In this process, the lungs play an essential role because they remove carbon dioxide from the blood and provide it with oxygen. Lung function declines remarkably as we age, seen as a decrease in both air flow and blood flow.

Aside from *seishin chousoku hou*, which I discussed in chapter 3, there are three ways to improve air flow. One involves focusing on and controlling breathing, while the other two require that you pay attention to strengthen the respiratory muscle in the chest and the abdomen.

In what I like to call the "separated breathing method," you should inhale deeply through the nose while silently counting to one. Count to two when exhaling through the nose and to three when inhaling again. Repeat this sequence of breathing through the nose until you exhale the air on the count of ten. Whenever I try this breathing method just before swimming, it enables me to swim underwater for a long period of time. Even Jacques Mayol, who was one of the most famous free divers, mentioned that we could improve the function of the lungs incredibly by controlling our breathing. Try it once a day.

You can make the respiratory muscle in your chest strong by breathing while simultaneously moving your arms in a flapping motion like a bird. (Flying birds are known to mainly breathe by moving both wings.) You should inhale deeply while raising your arms slowly and then exhale while lowering them slowly. You should do this in a sequence of ten once or twice a day, and all breathing should be done from the nose.

Squats are also effective when synchronized with breathing. This exercise will help strengthen abdominal muscles, but when you combine the squat with breathing, your respiratory muscle will also undergo amazing transformation, helping you to stay young and fit. This prisoner squat isn't very different from the traditional squat, but your movement should be synchronized to your breathing. First, standing with your feet hip-width apart and your hands behind your ears, and then stick your chest out, stretching the elbows back (Fig. 8). As you exhale, squat until your knees are bent as low as you can go without losing the arch of the spine (Fig. 9). Finally, push yourself back up to starting position as you inhale through the mouth. This exercise should be done in a sequence of ten once or twice a day. Of course, you shouldn't do this exercise if you have problems with your legs or knees.

As for blood flow in the lungs, even in healthy young people, there is a discrepancy between the upper and the lower portion of both lungs at standing position because of gravity. Such discrepancy will increase with age. However, if we do proper aerobic exercises, we can slow down this process. I maintain that walking is the best exercise of all because it is already a part of our daily routine and is easy to do anytime and anywhere. It is important that you maintain a rate of speed that allows you to breathe through the nose. Ideally, you should walk for over fifteen minutes several times a week.

Drinking plenty of water is important in improving blood flow as well. Unless we get an adequate supply, the blood flow will be too poor in the lungs to get enough oxygen into the body or clear the airways of mucous and phlegm. You should drink at least fifty-one ounces of water a day.

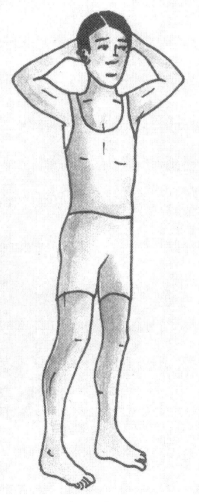

(Fig. 8)

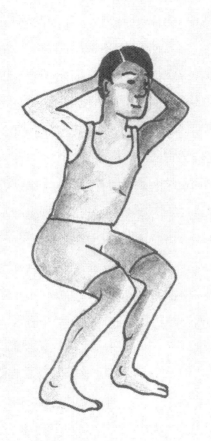

(Fig. 9)

Chapter 7: Eating Food and Cleaning the Colon

In developed countries, obesity, the result of a high-calorie diet, is a serious problem. Obesity is a risk factor for diabetes mellitus, heart disease, and stroke, all of which can be fatal. The rise in the consumption of drinks with high sugar content is alarming as a source of high-calorie. Unless you kick your liquid sugar habit, you would not live long.

In contrast, people in Japan tend to eat foods that are low in calories and high in antioxidants, both of which are factors in helping them live long, healthy lives. Antioxidants are effective in preventing tissue injuries by removing damaging free radicals, which speed up the aging process and can be carcinogenic. Foods such as green tea, soybeans, tomatoes, pumpkin, broccoli, parsley, eel, salmon, and red wine are all high in antioxidants. In addition to cutting calories, eating more of these foods is one key to living a longer life.

In maintaining your well-being, how you eat is just as important as what you eat. When you are eating, do you ever think about the food itself? For example, when you eat an apple, do you think about where or how it was grown? Before you got the apple, it might have been carefully grown by somebody at an orchard. At that time, the apple was alive like you! You should not take the apple for granted, because it is a gift from the soil. Recognizing this fact will help you to appreciate not only the food you eat but also lots of other people who help you. Through the food you eat you can see that you are living surrounded by both the blessing of nature and other people's help. Think about the food you eat. It could make a huge difference in your quality of life, and by doing so you will have the delightful knowledge that this food is truly the source of life. As a result, eating food will make you happy through this consideration.

The colon and its bacteria play an extremely important role in digesting this food. In the colon, we have numerous bacteria, which amount to just over two pounds of our body weight. Recently in Japan there has been a focus on cleaning the colon in order to stay young and fit. That is to say, people are trying to eat foods that increase the good bacteria in the colon and decrease the bad.

As we age, the good bacteria decrease and the bad bacteria increase. This change is one of the reasons why the elderly often get colon cancer. In order to stay healthy, we have to improve the environment in the colon. Fortunately, we can do this by taking in foods that contain good bacteria and high amounts of fiber. In addition, if we eat such foods daily, we can prevent obesity and decrease the level of bad cholesterol in the blood, both of which are terrible risk factors for heart attacks and strokes. It is also known that oligosaccharide, which is found in the soybean, supports the task of good bacteria in conjunction with fiber as feed for them.

Knowing this helps us to figure out what kinds of food we should eat to clean our colon. Yogurt is known to contain lots of good bacteria, known as lactobacillus. And in Japan, we regularly eat foods like miso soup, natto, and soy sauce, all of which are made from the fermented soybean, yet another source of lactobacillus. I believe that this Japanese dietary habit might contribute to our longevity. In addition, you should try to eat food that contains lots of fiber, such as oatmeal, mushrooms, seaweed, and vegetables like cabbage and broccoli.

If you take care of eating food as I mentioned here, you will end up finding an amazing way keeping you fit and youthful.

Summary of Practices and Exercises

- Look your face and whole body in a mirror to check your aging.

- Remember the ambitions and hopes of your youth to reconnect with the sense of strong vitality.

- Encourage and trust yourself through the thought that your existence and life is a miracle in the cosmos.

- Wrap your arms around a big tree and communicate with it in silence to bring about awareness of your soul.

- Lie on your back in bed and close your eyes in the dark. After that relax all of your muscles until you can't feel any weight in every part of your body. This practice should be done for about twenty minutes at least twice a week.

- Try to do the breathing of *seishin chousoku hou*. First, take a deep breath, feeling the air filling up and expanding your lungs. Second, hold your breath for one or two seconds as a slow transition. Third, exhale from your nose little by little. Finally, after exhaling, take a short breath. (You have to inhale and exhale through your nose.) This sequence of breathing may be done in either a sitting or lying position, but it should be done for more than ten minutes, once or twice a day, with your eyes closed and your hands clasped together resting on the lap.

- Do such meditation as below in combination with a breathing method, *seishin chousoku hou* in order to remind both the body and the mind of your youth. Imagine yourself listening to the songs that were popular when you were young while doing the breathing method, *seishin chousoku hou*. You need to actually listen to the music in your mind, without the aid of CDs or MP3s. This combination of breathing and meditation should be done continuously more than three times a week.

- While walking, pay attention to keep the lower central portion of your back as the center of your gravity to improve not only your walking posture but also athletic ability.

- Try to yawn intentionally as often as you can.

- Open your mouth and bridge either a chopstick a pencil between the corners of the mouth while sitting on a chair. (you should take care not to bite down on the chopstick or the pencil.)

- Lying on your back in bed, first turn your head to the right, stretching both the right arm and leg while bending the left arm and leg. Keep that position for five minutes. Then, turn your head to the left and repeat the exercise on the opposite side for another five minutes.

- Put the back of your right hand in your left palm. Then, put both hands under the head and lie in bed. After that bend the left leg, placing your foot over the right knee. Keep that position for five minutes. Then, putting the back of your left hand in your right palm, repeat this position on the opposite side for five minutes.

- Try sticking out your tongue and writing your name or a short sentence ("I'm fine and still young," for example) in the air, using only the tip of your tongue like a pen, and without moving your head.

- Move your eyes left and right, and up and down, as quickly as possible while you are looking at the sky without moving your head for fifteen seconds.

- Alternately turn your head back and forth to looking back over each shoulder while walking. At that time, you will have to move your eyes quickly to see both the right side and the left side alternately.

- Try to *kampumasatsu*. Rub the skin on all area of the body except for the head with a dry towel. You should take care not to rub the skin too hard. (Those suffering from a skin disease should avoid this practice.)

- Try to do "separated breathing method." First, inhale deeply through the nose while silently counting to one. Second, exhale a half of the air in the lungs counting one, and after holding breath for less than one second, exhale the rest of the air in the lungs counting to two. Third, inhale dividedly three times with two times breath holdings for less than one second counting to three until the lungs are completely expanded. Repeat this sequence of breathing until you exhale the air on the count of ten. Do this once a day.

- Inhale deeply while raising your arms slowly, and then exhale deeply while lowering them more slowly. Do this in a sequence of ten once or twice a day.

- Try to do the squats synchronized with breathing. First, standing with your feet hip-width apart and your hands behind your ears, and then stick your chest out, stretching the elbows back. As you exhale, squat until your knees are bent as low as you can go without losing the arch of the spine. Finally, push yourself back up to starting position as you inhale through the mouth. This exercise should be done in a sequence of ten once or twice a day. (Those having problems with their legs or knees should avoid this exercise.)

- Try to do walking as an aerobic exercise. Walk for over fifteen minutes several times a week. You should take care to both maintain a rate of speed that allows you to breathe through the nose and focus on keeping the lower central portion of your back as the center of your gravity while walking.

- Try to drink at least fifty-one ounces of water a day. (Those suffering from a heart disease, a renal disease, a hormonal disorder, and so on need to be allowed to do this by their doctors.)

- Try to eat foods that are low in calories and high in antioxidants.

- Think about the food that you are about to eat. As a result, you will get the delightful knowledge that you are living surrounded by both the blessing of nature and other people's help.

- Try to eat foods which contain lots of good bacteria and fiber in order to clean your colon.

References

Bryan, M., and K. Dorling. 2001. *The story of philosophy.* Penguin Group (USA): Penguin Books.

Chan, E. D., and C. H. Welsh.1998. Geriatric respiratory medicine. *Chest* 114: 1704-1733.

Ehrsam, R. E., et al. 1983. Influence of aging on pulmonary hemodynamics at rest during supine exercise. *Clinical Science* 65:653-660.

Gerd, G. 2007. *Gut feelings.* Penguin Group (USA): Penguin Books.

Haruto, I. 1992. Gakuhenishou. Tokyo: Justic Press.

Hiroshi, S., and Y. Hajime. 1978. *Breathing illustrated.* Tokyo: Takeda Pharmaceutical Company Limited.

Isao, S. 2009. Mechanisms underlying the aging process and anti-aging strategy. *Japan Journal of Clinical Medicine.* 67: 1265-1270.

Jacques, M. 1983. *Homo delphinus.* Florence: Giunti Martello.

Kiyoji, T., and M. Tomoaki. 2009. Effects of exercise and physical activity on real age. *Japan Journal of Clinical Medicine*. 67: 1361-1365.

Kouichirou, F. 2008. *Kiseichyuhakase no furou no menekigaku*. Tokyo: Koudansha Co.

Matsumoto, M., et al. 2001. Impact of LKM512 yogurt on improvement of intestinal environment of elderly. FEMS. *Immunological Medicine Microbiology*. 31: 181-186.

Masamichi, I., and Y. Makoto. 2009. Mitochondrial dysfunction as promoting factor of senescence. *Japan Journal of Clinical Medicine*. 67: 1321-1325.

Mikio, T., et al. 2001. *Kenkou to undou no kagaku*. Vol. 7. Tokyo: Taishunkanshoten Press.

Nobuo. S. 2007. *Daikenkouryoku*. Vol. 13. Tokyo: Golf Digest Co.

Norman, D. 2007. *The brain that changes itself*. Penguin Group (USA): Penguin Books.

Richard, Kraut. 2008. *How to read Plato*. London: Granta Books.

Ryuuichi, N., S. Hiroshi, and N. Hiroshi. 2006. *Fundamental kinesiology*. 5th ed. Tokyo: Ishiyaku Publishers, Inc.

Shin, F. 2007. *Naizou kankaku (Nou to chou no fushigina kankei)*. Nippon Housou Kyoukai. Tokyo: NHK Books.

Shunryu, S. 2002. *Not always so: Practicing the true spirit of Zen*. Ed. Edward E. Brown. New York: Harper Collins Publishers.

Simon, I. 2007. *The eye: A natural history*. London, New York, Berlin: Bloomsbury Publishing.

Tsuneo, M. 2008. *Chounaijouka kenkouhou*. Tokyo: PHP Researcher Press.

Turnbaugh, P. J., et al. 2006. An obesity-associated gut microbiome with increase capacity for energy harvest. *Nature* 444: 1027-1031.

Weisberg, H. F. 1962. *Water, electrolyte, and acid-base balance.* 2nd ed. Baltimore: Williams and Wilkins Co.

Yoshimi, B. 2008. *Chounai kankyou gaku.* Iwanamishoten. Tokyo: Iwanami Science Library.

Yoshio, H. 2000. *Kamiawase no kyoui.* Koudansha Co. Tokyo: Blue Backs.